3...2...1...

W. James Patrick

LOSE WEIGHT WITHOUT EXERCISE

The Information You Need

by W. James Patrick

W. James Patrick

Copyright © 2019

All Rights Reserved.

No part of this book may be reproduced without the expressed written consent of the publisher.

The publisher is not liable or responsible for any negative side affects or harm that the use or misuse of the practices within may cause to an individual reader. The reader bears responsibility for his or her body and must implement any advice in this book with caution and medical consultation if felt necessary. Not all bodies are the same and medical conditions and medications a person may have or take can complicate even straight forward good advice.

Table of Contents:

Introduction

Chapter 1: Why are you overweight?

Chapter 2: Your goals and vision for yourself

Chapter 3 Mistakes people make with weight loss and what really matters

Chapter 4 First steps to a new life

Chapter 5 What to eat and drink and why

Chapter 6 -Exercise

Conclusion

Introduction

Dear reader, thank you for buying this book as part of your quest for a healthier version of yourself. The first step to solving a problem is admitting there is one so you may not feel it just yet, but you have taken a big step towards the self improvement you want.

This book will contain information that you should see as tools to use on your journey as this truly is YOUR journey and the victory will be all yours. It is difficult to change too many things at once and we are all different so you are your own guide on how best to use the information here to get your body to where you want it to be

In this book I will discuss the problem of obesity in a holistic way so that different aspects of why people end up needing to lose weight can be brought to readers attention. This varies from person to person so it's best to attack the problem from all sides.

For some readers the underlying cause of being overweight may require help that is beyond the scope of this book whether it's a more serious physical or psychological condition.

This book is not a body positivity book where I will talk about how you should feel good and feel beautiful about being overweight. We would never tell an anorexic person on the verge of death from starvation that they are perfectly healthy as long as they are happy about it. Being overweight leads to many bad medical conditions so this book prioritises a heathy body over any other aspects of the discussion of peoples weight that we hear.

Chapter 1

Why are you overweight?

In my life I have known people who were overweight for different reasons. For some, I would give them dietary advice and they would implement it and over time and they would lose weight. Some of those would gain the weight back after more time. Some would remain at a lower weight. Other people I have known just couldn't implement any dietary plan whatsoever. Some of those people lived a lifestyle that made it awkward to be disciplined and others didn't really want to try at all. These people would say they want to lose weight but nothing about their behaviour looked like they really meant it. I've known other people who have lost nearly 100 pounds for an event in the future that they wanted to look good for and they would get down to their target weight, but then slowly over time they would gain a lot of it back. So asking you the question is very important — why are you overweight? Perhaps you will really need to think about that and be honest with yourself in a way thats new to you, but without truly knowing whats driving your lifestyle that leads you to being overweight it will be impossible to solve the problem in the long term.

A relative of mine was massively overweight. One evening in conversation she revealed to me that was gay. She's not from a family that has anything against gay people, but being secretly gay was a big problem for her. We are social animals that need to feel a connection to and feel accepted and approved by others for who we truly are, especially the people close to us. So for her, she had a massive problem over her head. If she told her parents she was gay and they didn't accept her for it, she would lose her relationship with her parents, but because they don't know who she truly is, the acceptance they have for her felt fake. She was 22 at the time and despite her fear and anxiety and plans to "never tell them" which then became "maybe next year," after two hours of persuading her why she was brave enough and why she was being selfish not giving her parents the chance to prove themselves to her, she came out to them that night.

The next time I saw her she looked like a different person. Just had a different aura to her. For her she felt "disgusting" being gay so allowing herself to be massively overweight didn't really matter to her. Once she had solved the problem of telling her parents she was gay and moved past that she was ready to deal with the weight problem.

Over the course of the next 14 months she lost 112 pounds. She found it easy. The comfort that eating bad foods gave her was gone. She still enjoys them from time to time and should lose another 20 pounds to get her weight down to what is ideal for her height, but she has transformed herself so much that she doesn't look fat anymore. Now that she is so much smaller, she was able to learn to drive which will give her many more opportunities which may include a new job, a new college course or a romantic relationship with someone who lives some distance from her town. I was very happy to be able to help her as I felt her life would have just been ruined had she stayed on the path she was on.

So using her as an example, it's easy to see why expecting her to lose weight, when it was only part of a bigger problem she had, was a bit unrealistic. We are only human so even if we can muster incredible willpower we can't do that in a sustained way in the longterm. It's best to solve a problem at its core so that we aren't swimming against the stream. You will have an idea for why you are overweight. It's worth really thinking about. Obviously it comes from eating too much of the wrong foods. Thats easily fixed. What's not so easily fixed is why you allow yourself to do that. The information that will follow in this book will help you transform yourself into the thin healthy version of yourself that you want. But before that can work for you, you will have to understand what is driving you to being overweight and solve that problem. Perhaps it is stress from some aspect of life, an unresolved relationship issue with someone close to you, perhaps you are truly uninformed as to how different foods affect the body, perhaps you live a lifestyle where the easy option is to eat stuff you know is bad for you. Life is not easy and nobody is spared from suffering and many of those people use alcohol, work, sex, money or food as a comfort. I wont be able to help you with an individual problem you might have but I can say that if you promise yourself you will tell the truth as you see it, and bring that honesty into the relationships with you with friends and family, and seek to uplift others when you can, thats the most you can do to create conditions where just being you is comfort enough from life's hardships.

Chapter 2

Your goals and vision for yourself

Although people say the journey is more important than the destination, that is not always the case. When it comes to weight loss you should know what you are aiming at. So what do you picture when you see your future-self who is in good physical shape? And don't limit your thinking here. Many of the people who are super-athletes were once very obese. As you allow yourself to fantasise about your future self who is thin and healthy, what do you see? For some people they want to be thin for a certain occasion, a wedding, a holiday, etc. Other people want to be able to wear certain types of clothing, or look good with clothes off. Perhaps you see yourself enjoying a more active lifestyle, appearing more put together in your professional or romantic life or maybe you'd be happy with just being more physically comfortable in your body. Being honest with yourself here is important. You need a destination in mind.

As important as knowing what you want is knowing what you don't want. Take a moment to think about what your life would be like in the future if you don't get control of your weight. Think about how bad it could get. Diseases and illness are all much more likely to happen to you if you are overweight. Do you really want to bring all that on yourself?

At this stage id like to invite you to think about items the future thin and healthy version of you might own. Perhaps a certain item of clothing or athletic gear. If an item comes to mind I recommend that you buy that item. The fact that you thought of it when I asked shows that it's a powerful item symbolically for you. Having it in your possession shows intent to yourself that you are serious about continuing your transformation. I'm not recommending you buy something expensive, even the smallest item that symbolises your future better self can be very powerful.

Chapter 3

Mistakes people make with weight loss and what really matters

Before we get to the actual tools and strategies you can use to transform your body and maybe even your life, I'd like to talk about what weight loss can be so confusing and hard for people.

The first thing is people have underlying issues that need to be addressed as I discussed earlier.

The second thing is that when they are truly ready to lose weight, they try to change too many things at once. I recommend only changing one thing a week. Perhaps you are someone who feels comfortable moving faster than that and you should move faster then. It only takes 3 weeks for a new behaviour to become a habit. This is important to know. Establishing new positive habits is what leads to success in the long run and makes the process feeling quite natural and easy.

The third thing people get wrong is that they think they can exercise fat away. Our bodies are so efficient at moving that we have to do so much exercise to burn enough calories to lose lots of weight that its just not sustainable. Even people who get themselves into good shape who allow themselves to eat poorly and think they can exercise enough to make up for that — the just end up gaining the weight back. Exercise has many positive aspects to it but it's not helpful to think it should to be used to fight fat. The rule of thumb is to understand you can't compensate for a bad diet with exercise. It's very difficult for people who are trying to get in shape and are overweight to change their diet and start exercising. The soreness and lack of visible results leads to the person just giving up within a few weeks. It's not the ideal strategy. Exercising when you are ready for it has many benefits. You will look better, feel better, it protects your health, improves your posture, makes your bones stronger, reduces stress, can be a social experience and with only a few intense minutes spent can protect your brain and level of intelligence from deteriorating with a process called neurogenesis where your body creates new brain cells. That alone is the case for why exercising is beneficial and is the main motivation for why I exercise. But as I said it's just not helpful for losing weigh to think of exercise being the way to do it. It can actually hurt the weight loss process for most people especially early on.

The fourth thing people get wrong about losing weight is thinking of the word diet as meaning "lack of food." This is not the case. Everyone is on a diet. You are either on a weight loss diet, a weight maintenance diet or a weight gain diet. It all just depends on the quantities of what foods you are eating. You can be on a weight gain diet and be hungry most of the time. You can be on a weight loss or maintenance diet and feel satisfied if not overfull. It all depends on how you use food. The correct outlook to have on this weight loss plan is that you are going to eat your way to being thin! There are foods you can eat that are very satisfying that burn off half their own calories to digest themselves and there are other foods that create a chemical reaction in your body that make you store fat and make you hungry again an hour after eating them. This is the information we all need.

Now, on to strategies.

Chapter 4

First steps to a new life

Step 1: The first step I recommend you take is that you look at your own diet as it is now. What are the foods you recognise as being bad for you that don't really give you that much pleasure? What are the top one or two things that you truly enjoy? People think they love chocolate or ice cream but in reality is only one particular type they ever have. It's important that you recognise what it is that you actually enjoy that you know is making you overweight so you can be very precise about what it is you might be crave. So the first step is identify the foods you really enjoy and notice how small the portion can be to satisfy you. People who slip up in their weight loss plan end up eating whole tubs of ice cream or entire 16 inch pizzas when they wouldn't do that even when they were comfort eating in an out of control manner. The first step is to become aware of how exactly you are eating. Try reducing servings of the unhealthy foods you enjoy and just notice how you feel. Try that for one week or sooner if you feel ready to move to step 2.

Step 2: is another very easy one. All you are going to do is eat all the food you are going to eat in a day inside of a 9 hour window. So say you start eating at 8am, at 5pm you stop eating until 8am the next day. The benefit of this is that it gives your body 15 hours to not have to metabolise food. Inside of that 15 hour window of fasting I recommend only having water or tea or coffee. Ideally only water but if you are a tea or coffee drinker, its ok to have some. This 15 hour fast period has many advantages. Eating inside of the 9 hour window and having 15 hours off is called intermittent fasting. Many professional athletes eat this way and train before they eat as they feel they perform better in the fasted state.Try it and see how you feel. You need to only imagine our ancestors and how they might go days without food and how we are shaped by that. We already fast hence the word "breakfast" but I recommend your breakfast, your first meal of the day, come after a 15 hour fast. If you are hungry during the 15 hours you need to ask yourself why you didn't eat what you needed in the 9 hour window.

People who live a lifestyle where they regularly eat for longer than a 12 hour window are much more likely to get diseases like cancer. A 12 hour eating window is the maximum I'd recommend, but a 9 hour window is the ideal. Try it for a week while keeping in mind what I talked about in step 1. If you are ready to improve your body faster then move at a faster pace.

Step 3: As I said at the start of this book, this is your journey. So far all I've recommended you do is bring a heightened awareness to how you use, eat and enjoy food. I will go into what foods I recommend you eat later, but so far you will have been using your own conscience and instincts and taking responsibility for yourself. I've also said to eat all your food inside of a 9 hour window, fast for 15 hours and repeat. How did you find that? It really doesn't require much discipline. If you are eating in a way for 9 hours that fails to satisfy you for the next 15 hours (including sleep) then perhaps it is the type of food you are eating. What's the point eating food that doesn't satisfy your hunger. We will get into the different types of food soon. In step 3 I want to tell you about something thats called thermogenesis. This is where the body generates heat. In the human body our blood runs quite hot, so much so that 75% of the calories we burn are just from keeping our blood warm. So, by that logic, if we lower our body temperature we will have to generate more heat and burn up calories and fat to do that. The easiest ways to do this are a, to sleep without a blanket with lowered air temperature from a window open or colder air conditioning if you can sleep like that or b, you could do the cold shower technique. What you do is you have a shower like you regularly do, but at the end turn the water to cold and let the water hit you between your shoulders on your back. This is unpleasant for about 4 seconds and after that it's fine. Stay there for about 2 minutes. This is a good chance to learn how much control your mind has over your body. Exposure to heat like from a sauna or cold like a cold shower are positive stresses on the body like exercise is. Doing this has many benefits to the body, but for the purpose of this book, the weight loss benefit is most important. We store something known as "brown fat" on our back between our shoulders and lowering the temperature there with cold water triggers thermogenesis in the body and this triggers fat burning. Try this for a week while continuing what you've been doing from steps 1 and 2 and see how you do. If the cold exposure is really not for you thats fine, but realise its a very useful tool and if you can handle it then that's great. This is your journey and its about what you really want.

Chapter 5

What to eat and drink and why

It is so tempting to just write, "Only eat meat and vegetables" and have that as the entire content of the chapter because that is what it boils down to. If you were to follow that advice you would eat yourself to being thin in a few months and notice results straight away. If it's not meat or a vegetable — don't eat it. I will explain in more detail.

The world of food is a complex one. Even terminology can be overlapping. For instance because tomatoes are a fruit and potatoes are a vegetable one can argue a serving of pizza and french fries are part of their RDA of fruit and vegetables. I am not going to complicate this section with details that I think end up just being counterproductive to most peoples goals. Another aspect of how complex food can be is that some vegetables lose some health benefits when cooked but also again other benefits that they don't have raw. Trying to navigate to having the perfect diet involves too many decisions for most people so they just end up eating whatever they want. That's why the "Only eat meat and vegetables" really does simplify things.

Lets look at the different food types you should keep in mind when asking yourself "should I eat this?". There are carbohydrates which are bread, rice, pasta, potatoes, cereals, pastries, If you want to lose weight you should avoid these.The big problem with these foods is they raise your insulin levels which not only makes you store fat, but also just makes you hungry again an hour or so later. If you absolutely must have bread then only have wholemeal bread. See this can be a slippery slope for people. They will think, "I know I shouldn't have bread but I can have wholemeal bread therefore how bad is normal white bread?" People who play that sort of game thinking they can outsmart the reality are just being foolish, but if not having bread is a make or break the diet thing for you then have wholemeal bread. Another thing that you can have, are sweet potatoes. It's the same type scenario as with the wholemeal bread, if you absolutely must have something like potatoes then have sweet potatoes.

The category of protein has meat and fish in it. You can eat as much of these as you want. This also includes eggs, chick peas, lentils, nuts and beans. The main part of sticking to this diet plan is not being hungry so you need to satisfy yourself with food that will do the job. These foods can be quite delicious so you should look forward to your meals and feel satisfied for hours after.

Dairy is another category where you could ruin your diet if you want by outsmarting yourself. In this diet plan you are allowed cheese, butter, milk and creme for your tea and coffee. If you end up thinking, "I am allowed cheese and butter which are from milk and chocolate and ice cream are also from milk, so I can have them too" you will be fooling only yourself.

Vegetables: eat as much of these as you want. Some are better than others, but as long as you are avoiding potatoes then you can eat as many vegetables as you want. We are learning all the time how crucial eating fibre is to our health and vegetables are a great source of fibre. If you struggle to eat vegetables then you can put them in a blender and drink them in seconds. The benefits of blending them are you don't have to cook them, you get to eat them raw without having to taste or chew them, you barely have to clean up after and you are getting more nutrition than most people who actually eat vegetables get. It may not taste great but what I like to put in my green smoothie are broccoli, spinach, kale, a carrot, avocado, a tomato and blueberries.

Salads, you can eat as much salad as you want, with minimal dressing though.

Sugar should be avoided as much as possible. It's so harmful to the body and raises insulin so high that it leads to more fat storage, more hunger and eventually illnesses like diabetes. Obviously eating things like ice cream are part of enjoying life so I'm not say-ing, "never eat sugar" — which many health advisers do say, but avoid sugar when you are a weight loss diet. When you do allow yourself to have sugary things like chocolate, ice cream and fizzy drinks, do so in small portions. If you absolutely have to have something sweet then one or two pieces of high percentage dark chocolate is allowed. Try to save your allowance of dark choc-olate until later in the day so you have it to look forward to and it will minimise temptation.

Fruits are a tricky one. We all think of fruit as being good for us and they are, but they also contain lots of sugar. So while I recom-mend blueberries, tomatoes and avocado, I wouldn't recommend you eat foods in the category of fruit without really thinking about it. Some people recommend you never eat fruit, but I don't agree.

You can eat as many mushrooms as you like.

I also recommend using garlic, ginger, curcumin and turmeric whenever you can.

I am not going to include sample meal plans because in my ex-perience this robs people of their sense of adventure and owner-ship of their new eating plan. I have given you the information you need as a guide, but you still have to figure out it all applies to you based on what you are like as an individual. Once you are the one to make the rules, you will follow them.

When it comes to what to drink, I recommend only water. Most people are either tea or coffee drinks so that is also allowed as part of this diet. You definitely want to avoid sugary drinks in-cluding fruit juices. In terms of alcohol you definitely want to go with lighter beers.

Chapter 6

Exercise

This book is about losing weight without exercising. The information I have provided you with up until this point will help you achieve that goal. In this chapter I want to give you information on exercising so that as you enjoy the new thin you and further your healthy lifestyle, you know some things that can be helpful. The priority is for you follow the steps in the earlier chapters until you are light enough to be able to exercise without it hurting your main weight loss strategies, but if you can implement these exercises and not change your strategies from the earlier chapters then you can do that. You may need to talk to your doctor based on how big you may be.

As I said earlier there are many benefits to exercise and it can be done very fast. The whole idea of hours in the gym just to be fit is nonsense. People who enjoy going to the gym for hours, good for them, but it's not necessary to exercise well. The level of intensity you have when exercising is what's most important and you can have a great workout in 2 or 3 minutes.

In order to maintain a strong mobile body you have to move. The gym, exercising, fitness classes, it's all just moving. You should never feel intimidated by the thought of joining a fitness club or class. Its just moving and its important to keep your body able to move. Plus everyone in those gyms and classes is too obsessed and worried about their own body and performance to even notice yours.

Sometimes it's hard to distinguish between exercise and just play, like games like tennis or golf. Even sex requires a level of stamina and mobility to be fun. So being physically fit is important for maximising your enjoyment of your life. The information in the world of fitness is very complex and even contradictory. This is done to make money. They want you paying for gym memberships and expensive equipment. All you really need is the floor and your own body weigh to give yourself a good workout.

If you are someone who is very heavy and can't move much I recommend you stand rather than sit. Stand as much as you can. This will rebuild your body and burn a lot of calories. In the USA, childhood obesity would not exist if children had standing desks in school. Never underestimate the power of walking. While it's not the cardio workout that running is, it is worthwhile to walk a lot. We are designed to walk a lot everyday.

There are a few different ways that your body needs to be fit.

The first type of fitness is your heart and lung conditioning. This is cardio. There are bodybuilders who have 4% body fat and massive muscles but get out of breath walking up stairs. That is not good. Any exercise that makes you breathe hard and makes your heart beat fast is cardio exercise. Running and cycling are examples. It is better to do it as hard as you can rather than a slow jog or light cycle if you are doing it to train your heart and lungs. Of course, doing anything is better than doing nothing.

The second type of fitness is your muscle strength. This is what lifting weights and resistant training is about. So say you are lifting weights, the purpose here is to train the muscles you are targeting rather than your heart and lungs. You should always know what the purpose of a particular exercise is. If you want to train a muscle, focus on that, if you want to exercise your heart and lungs, then focus on that. While the two types of fitness can overlap a little, they don't always. I know people who lift weights four times a week but couldn't run half a mile and there are others who can run 30 miles but have weak legs.

I am going to give you a beginners workout routine that you should be able to complete in minutes. It is to get you started and you can then explore all that is on offer in the world of fitness from yoga classes to weight lifting to cycling. There are many options and once you have your weight under control you will see fitness activities as forms of fun.

The things to keep in mind about exercise is that it's good for brain. This is achieved by causing neurogenesis which is a by-product of putting a positive stress on the body. This means running to your maximum and making your muscles burn from lifting weights to the maximum you can. This can take only a few seconds. Here are the two workout routines I recommend for you as a beginner. Also, when doing these exercises, only breathe in and out through your nose. Mouth breathing feels like its bigger breathing because your mouth is bigger than your nostrils, but when you stick to only breathing through your nose, it keeps your diaphragm's breathing rhythm intact and is more efficient.

Routine 1: Sprints

You will need to be in a place where you can run your fastest for 20 seconds in a straight line. You can do this on a treadmill too but its easy to do it on grass as well. So all you do is walk and then run as fast as you can for 20 seconds and then walk for 90 seconds and then sprint again for 20 seconds as fast you can. Repeat until you have done 3 sprints. This trains your heart and lungs at maximum capacity. This is so much better than going out and jogging at mild pace for an hour. Do this at least once a week but aim for twice.

Routine 2: Squats and Push Ups

With this one you are going to alternate between squats and push ups. You will do one squat and then one push up. Then two squats and then two push ups. The fact you are dropping down to the ground and getting back up is part of the exercise too. Keep repeating and increasing the number and watch how you improve. Make sure to do the squats and push ups slowly and because it is such a full body workout you will breathing heavy too. Do this at least once a week but do it twice if you can leaving 3 days between them.

I'm quite an expert on fitness, but what I have written there is all you really need to get you in great shape. I could give you a workout routine that takes 2 hours a day in the gym with different techniques for moving weights around and stretching, but most people don't want to spend that much time exercising. The workout routines I have given you here, if you do them with proper intensity, you would complete them in way less than 10 minutes. A tip to help you find that time is to notice when the clock is less than 20 minutes before the next hour and challenge yourself to get the workout done before the new hour.

Conclusion

I hope this information helps you on your journey and that you achieve what you want to achieve. It's not rocket science. If you'd like you can share your progress in the review section. I look forward to reading about of your happiness and success. I hope my book will be beneficial to you. Best of luck.